Alcohol Addiction: How to Stop Drinking and Recover from Alcohol Addiction

The following Book is reproduced below with the goal of providing information that is as accurate and reliable as possible. Regardless, purchasing this Book can be seen as consent to the fact that both the publisher and the author of this book are in no way experts on the topics discussed within and that any recommendations or suggestions that are made herein are for entertainment purposes only. Professionals should be consulted as needed prior to undertaking any of the action endorsed herein.

This declaration is deemed fair and valid by both the American Bar Association and the Committee of Publishers Association and is legally binding throughout the United States.

Furthermore, the transmission, duplication, or reproduction of any of the following work including specific information will be considered an illegal act irrespective of if it is done electronically or in print. This extends to creating a secondary or tertiary copy of the work or a recorded copy and is only allowed with the express written consent from the Publisher. All additional rights reserved.

The information in the following pages is broadly considered a truthful and accurate account of facts and as such, any inattention, use, or misuse of the information in question by the reader will render any resulting actions solely under their purview. There are no scenarios in which the publisher or the original author of this work can be in any fashion deemed liable for any hardship or damages that may befall them after undertaking information described herein.

Additionally, the information in the following pages is intended only for informational purposes and should thus be thought of as universal. As befitting its nature, it is presented without assurance regarding its prolonged validity or interim quality. Trademarks that are mentioned are done without written consent and can in no way be considered an endorsement from the trademark holder.

Table of Contents

BONUS:

As a way of saying thank you for purchasing my book, please use your link below to claim your free ebook

I have laid down Top 10 Tips Guide for you to Overcoming Obsessions and Compulsions Using Mindfulness

https://bit.ly/2TDMNkn

You can also share your link with your friends and families whom you think that can benefit from the guide or you can forward them the link as a gift!

Introduction

Alcoholism is an extreme dependency on consuming alcohol in order to be able to function in society. It also refers to the illnesses of the mind and the extreme behavioral compulsions that are a direct effect of drinking to excess. Alcoholism is a continuous excessive disease that is identifiable by compulsively drinking alcoholic beverages to excess. This practice leads to physical and psychological addiction or dependence. People who are alcoholics are unable to control their drinking. They have no real control over the need to drink often and excessively. This tendency often displays as an inability to go to work regularly or to perform properly when at work. Alcoholics will either socialize way too much or will be unable to socialize with others. Many alcoholics prefer to drink alone, not only because it is quieter and they can focus on the drink but also so there are no other people to judge how much they drink.

Alcoholics are often characterized by their slovenly appearance. When alcoholism takes over most people eventually stop bathing regularly and no longer care about their personal appearance. They do not cut or wash their hair. They do not change clothes regularly, and their clothing is often food-stained and reeking of human body odor. Some alcoholics display violent tendencies. The most mild-mannered person in the world can become a vicious beast or a raving lunatic when the alcohol takes over their senses.

People who are alcoholics are susceptible to certain diseases that do not regularly affect the general public. Alcoholics have an increased risk of developing hepatitis, an inflammation of the tissue in the liver. They are also most likely to suffer from cirrhosis of the liver, which is scarring of the tissue due to the effects of other illnesses that affect the liver. Alcoholics also have an increased risk of developing alcohol poisoning due to the fact that alcoholic beverages are consumed rapidly in a short amount of time.

Alcoholism knows no boundaries. Anyone, anywhere, at any time, can become an alcoholic. It knows no age limit, nor does it prefer one gender over another. Alcoholism does not care if you are rich or you are poor. Alcoholism has been a public health crisis for many generations. This is an amazing fact considering that only about half the people in the world consume all of the alcohol. There are many countries in the world where almost no one drinks any form of alcohol due to religious reasons.

Part of the problem, and part of the reason that alcoholism can so easily become a problem is that alcohol is everywhere. In most towns and cities it is impossible to drive down the street without passing a liquor store, a bar, or a club. Many large cities even advertise their more popular bars. Alcohol can be found at many activities, and many activities grew up around the consumption of alcohol. Consider the college campus and happy hour at the bar. Think of the Friday night mixers and the BYOB (Bring Your Own Bottle) reminder where the host or hostess supplied various mixers. And there are always the holiday gatherings, where even multi-generational families will toast the New Year with a glass of champagne.

So alcoholism does not care where people come from, what they believe, or what they do for a living. Alcoholism is a disease that strikes where it feels like striking and when it feels like striking. Sometimes whole families are alcoholics, and sometimes it is one person in a family of teetotalers. Sometimes one or both parents are alcoholics, but the children never touch a drop. Sometimes the parents do not drink at all, or only socially, and the children become alcoholics. Alcoholics are college graduates and high school dropouts. Alcoholics have jobs and children. Alcoholics drive on the same roads as everyone else.

Numerous negative effects are caused by alcoholism that wreak havoc on the human body. No area of the body is immune to the negative effects of too much drinking. And anyone of these effects has the potential to be life-altering or even deadly.

The communication paths in the brain can be seriously affected by drinking too much. The pathways in the brain control the travel of conscious thought and are created by constantly thinking a thought or practicing a habit. Alcohol can disrupt these pathways and cause differences in the way the brain thinks and reacts to stimuli. It can also create changes in behavior and overall mood. The ability to clearly think and move with grace and ease may be affected.

Excessive drinking can damage the heart. The first effect of drinking on the body is usually a rise in blood pressure to a level that is considered dangerous. Strokes are a direct cause of high blood pressure. Excessive drinking is also responsible for cardiac arrhythmias, where the heart does not beat at a regular pace but suffers irregular beats. This can cause a heart attack. Perhaps the worst effect on the heart is a disease called cardiomyopathy, which is characterized by malformation of the heart muscle that includes drooping or stretching. This physical irregularity can lead to complete heart failure.

The liver is another organ that is directly affected by too much drinking. Once the liver becomes inflamed from too much drinking, the person is at a greater risk of developing hepatitis that may not be curable because of the inflammation of the liver. Excessive drinking can also lead to a condition called fatty liver, where excess fat becomes stored in the liver, and the liver finds it difficult to remove this excess fat because it has suffered damage. Possibly the worst damage to the liver is a disease called cirrhosis which is abnormal scarring of the liver that cannot be replaced by normal liver regeneration. When cirrhosis is involved the only cure is a transplant of a healthy liver.

Most people forget that the effects of alcoholism can also damage the pancreas. The pancreas is the organ that secretes digestive juices into the small intestine to aid in digestion. The pancreas is also responsible for the production and secretion of insulin into the bloodstream. Insulin is the chemical in the body that controls blood sugar.

Besides the enormous health problems that are associated with alcoholism, there are also problems associated with behavior that can harm the drinking person. People who are inebriated often have no fear and might find themselves in dangerous situations. They may try to fight other people. They may engage in harmful activities such as climbing high structures or walking where it might be dangerous. Driving is the worst thing a drunk person can do because they risk not only their own lives but the lives of others. Alcoholism is a dangerous condition that can have many negative effects on the human body, and consequently, on life itself.

Chapter 1: Alcohol Addiction and Health Challenges

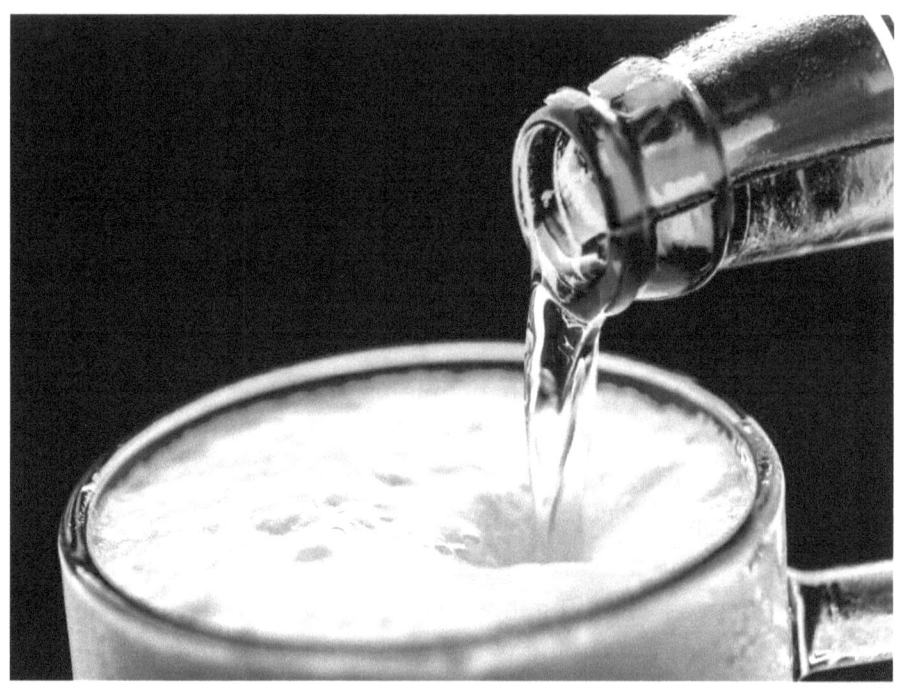

Alcoholism, also known as alcohol addiction, affects people in any area of life. Many experts have studied alcoholics looking for a common factor of what might lead to alcoholism. But alcohol addiction does not care if a person is a male or female, rich or poor, or what color they are or what religion they follow. Unfortunately, no one factor predisposes someone to become an alcoholic. It has no main cause. Behavioral, genetic, and psychological factors all have a contribution to someone developing alcohol addiction.

Alcoholism is a disease. Some people may argue that it is simply a lack of will power, that alcoholics are weak-willed and could quit on their own if they tried hard enough. But this is not the case with alcohol addiction. The excess drinking that causes alcoholism leads to negative changes in the chemistry of the brain. A person who has alcohol addiction may truly be unable to control their own actions.

Alcoholism shows up in various ways. The disease differs in severity between people, how often they drink, and how much they drink. Some people only drink after work is done for the day. Some people drink for several days and then stay sober for a short period. Some people drink heavily throughout the entire day.

The key to alcohol addiction is not the pattern of drinking. The key is that the person is unable to stay sober for more than a short period of time and the person must eventually rely on alcohol to be able to function with some normalcy.

The symptoms of alcohol addiction can be difficult to pinpoint in the individual. Since alcohol is readily available and such a part of many celebrations it is widely considered a socially acceptable beverage. Therefore it may be difficult to know, at least in the beginning, that someone has a problem with alcohol consumption. Society has become adept at turning a blind eye to someone who might have a drinking problem.

Many signs might point to alcohol addiction. Obviously, people with a drinking problem drink much more and much more often than people who do not have a drinking problem. This will give them a higher tolerance than most people, meaning they will need to drink more to feel the effects of the alcohol. Alcoholics often do not have hangovers, perhaps because they are never truly sober. Alcoholics will usually drink at times that other people consider inappropriate. Alcoholics may feel the need to drink as soon as they get out of bed, or they may drink over lunch at work. People with an alcohol addiction do not want to go where there will not be alcohol offered. Those who have an alcohol addiction may leave old friends behind in favor of new, heavy drinking buddies. They will begin to avoid loved ones, and may even lie to them about how much they really drink. They will hide their alcohol, so they always have a secret stash available. Alcoholics have even been known to hide while drinking, such as spending more time than might be necessary in the bathroom or the laundry room. As the disease progresses, the alcoholic will become increasingly dependent on alcohol just to be able to make it through the day. They will begin to experience emotional issues such as depression or extreme anger and will suffer from excessive lethargy. Alcoholics often experience legal problems that come with being arrested for public drunkenness or driving while intoxicated. They may also face demotions at work or even job loss.

Consumption of excessive amounts of alcohol creates effects on the brain that may explain why some people become alcoholics. When people drink the chemical balance in the brain is altered. Alcohol is a downer, a depressant, and it is an attractive legal drug to people who suffer from extreme stress, depression, or a lowered sense of self-worth. After just one drink a person can become much less anxious and much more self-confident. The alcohol lowers the chemical makeup in the part of the brain that has to do with inhibiting feelings. People build a deep desire to drink more alcohol in order to increase positive feelings and reduce the negative ones. This deep desire becomes a craving that can eventually lead to alcoholism.

Unfortunately, genetics may play an important role in deciding who becomes an alcoholic and who does not. Children who grow up with alcoholics are much more likely to become alcoholics themselves. This may also be due to other factors in the environment the child is raised in, but it is believed that genetics has a part in alcohol addiction.

When people speak of environmental factors that may contribute to alcoholism, there are several. Alcohol is available almost anywhere, even in the grocery store or the gas station. People are more likely to drink if people around them are drinking. Alcohol advertisement is everywhere because drinking is supposed to be cool. Drinking is said to elevate a person's status socially. Happy people go to parties and drink a lot.

Alcoholics can suffer from a number of alcohol-related health problems that may or may not be treatable. Frequently consuming too much alcohol can have a negative effect on nearly every system in the body. When someone consumes more alcohol than the body is able to metabolize, the excess is funneled to the bloodstream. The heart will then continuously circulate the alcohol through the body in an effort to locate a place to store it. This leads to changes in the chemistry of the body and affects normal functions of the body.

The body metabolizes most of the alcohol it consumes in the liver. This is why the liver typically suffers so much damage as a result of alcoholism. In the liver, alcohol is changed into a toxic chemical that is known to cause cancer. Excessive drinking causes excess fat to build up in the body, causing a decrease in normal function in the liver. The liver can easily become inflamed, making the body more likely to develop hepatitis. And the increased strain on the liver causes a condition known as cirrhosis, which is scarring in the liver caused by all the other bad effects of alcohol consumption on the liver.

The pancreas, which is the organ responsible for supplying insulin to the body, can also be damaged by excessive and long-term effects of alcohol consumption. The pancreas can become inflamed, and a long period of inflammation can lead to pancreatic cancer.

Chronic excessive consumption of excessive amounts of alcohol can cause an increase in the risk of developing different types of cancer, including cancer of the breast, larynx, stomach, liver, rectum, colon, esophagus, and mouth.

Too much drinking will weaken the function of the immune system. Decreased immunity makes the body vulnerable to many diseases that are caused by infections such as tuberculosis and pneumonia. If these are contracted by a heavy drinker, it will be more difficult for them to recover quickly, if at all, due to their weakened immune systems.

Excessive alcohol consumption causes brain damage. It is the cause of slower reactions, lapses in memory, problems when walking, speech problems such as slurring words or a need to search for words, and vision problems like blurring or double vision. Alcoholics are often injured in falls that happen when they have been drinking because they stumble or are having difficulty seeing obstacles.

People who drink to excess regularly often suffer from poor nourishment and a deficiency in vitamins the body needs to function properly. Alcoholics usually have bad dietary habits. Nutrients from food are not used properly by the body due to reduced function of the gastrointestinal tract. Cells in the body, damaged by the constant onslaught of alcohol, are unable to absorb nutrients properly. The lining of the stomach may break down and begin to bleed, causing poor absorption of nutrients.

Osteoporosis leads to an increased risk of bone breakage and arthritis. Alcohol consumption disrupts the body's ability to absorb vitamin D and calcium, which leads to a drastic weakness in the structure of the bones. Those who drink to excess are more likely to suffer from broken bones than people who do not drink to excess. This is even truer when teens and young adults drink excessively. They can cause changes in the bone structure of the body that will lead to osteoporosis in later years, even if no other risk factors for osteoporosis are present.

Heavy alcohol consumption causes high blood pressure which can lead to strokes. Alcoholics have an increased risk of developing heart failure due to the increased workload the heart suffers trying to filter the excess alcohol out of the body.

Any amount of alcohol consumption can lead to an increase in accidents. Alcoholics often suffer from domestic violence, car wrecks, accidental drownings, slips and falls, and suicide than people who are not alcoholics.

Numerous health benefits will be experienced when a person quits drinking. The first benefit is just a better overall feeling. Without having to constantly process an overabundance of alcohol the body will begin to cleanse itself. The systems in the body regain their natural function and begin to function more closely to normal. The body is no longer required to process so many toxins so it can use that energy for other things. The mind also begins to function better. The mind will be clearer and more focused. Thoughts will be well-focused and will make more sense. The skin will begin to look better, softer and more youthful. Previous skin irritations will begin to clear. Alcohol causes the body to dehydrate, and a lack of hydration causes the skin to dry out and look older. Excessive alcohol consumption also causes the skin on the face to look red because tiny blood vessels break due to high blood pressure. The cells of the body will also function more efficiently. They will be better able to absorb vitamins and nutrients which will make the body healthier overall. Alcohol is a high-calorie drink. People who quit drinking often find they will easily lose weight. And since the alcohol calories are completely devoid of nutrients, replacing them with nutritious foods gives the body access to more natural vitamins. The heart will be healthier. The liver will be cleaner and will enjoy better function.

There are other benefits associated with quitting drinking. Sober people are better able to make connections with other people. Sobriety brings about a renewed desire to connect with friends and relatives, relationships that may have been neglected in favor of a night spent with alcohol. Drinking causes isolation and aloneness. It is more natural to want to connect with other people than it is to connect with alcohol. People who quit drinking will have more time to reconnect with a forgotten hobby or even to learn a new one. Drinking is time-consuming. It takes a lot of time away from more productive activities. Sober people find it easier to sleep better and more regularly. People who quit drinking find it easier to focus and be alert.

Alcoholism is a horribly debilitating disease. It causes massive health problems that can lead to great disability or even early death. It causes numerous mental health problems. Alcoholism not only ruins normal life, but it also takes the place of normal life. Making the decision to quit, and following through, will bring wonderful benefits to the body and the mind, and will enable a return to a more meaningful, fulfilling life.

Chapter 2: How Alcoholism Begins

Alcoholism is a disease marked by the impairment caused by constant and excessive consumption of alcohol. This impairment can directly cause physiological, social, or psychological dysfunction. Alcoholism is not just about how much a person drinks. Many people drink to excess on occasion and are not alcoholics. Alcoholism is more a function of how the alcohol affects the person. If drinking causes other problems in life, then there is a good chance that person is an alcoholic. Unfortunately, alcoholism has become a common disease.

Alcohol addiction often starts quite innocently. People do not start with the idea of being an alcoholic. Alcohol is a drink readily available at many social functions. People gather to drink a few drinks and share good times. The problem starts when people, having seen how good a few drinks made them feel at the party last week, take a drink to relieve the stress of a long work day. Whenever someone begins drinking to relieve stress, or to mask any other problem, they are setting a dangerous precedent. Because once alcohol is used as a problem solver or a problem masker, the stage is set for the beginning of alcoholism.

Being able to understand how alcohol addiction begins and how it develops can make it easier to realize when there is a problem with oneself or a loved one. Knowing how alcoholism works makes it easier to fight against.

In the early stages of alcoholism, people begin to have negative experiences that are directly related to excess drinking. These negative experiences include blackouts, violence toward other people, arguments with those closest to them, and hangovers. A hangover is an aftereffect of too much drinking the night before. It is marked by headache, fatigue, excessive thirst, dry mouth, and nausea. A blackout is just what it says it is: the person drinking has blacked out the memory of the time they were drinking. They have little to no memory of the night before. During the early stage of alcoholism, people notice their tolerance is increasing. They must constantly drink more and more alcohol to get the same good feeling they did before. They may begin to seek out new locations to drink and new people to drink with, so no one will know exactly how much they are really drinking.

In the middle stage of alcoholism, life begins to unravel. The person starts to lose control of their life. They will usually deny that any kind of problem exists. But now the person is drinking more than they were before. In this stage, the addiction is firmly set. People who try to stop drinking without outside help are often not successful. Work life may begin to slide downhill, and personal life offers more problems than solutions. They may begin to treat the morning hangover with an early drink, a little 'hair of the dog.' Also in this stage, the person begins to experience depression or anxiety. And even the presence of problems directly associated with drinking, like legal problems or emotional and physical problems are not enough to make them stop drinking.

Anyone who drinks long enough will eventually reach the last stage of alcoholism. In this stage, the person has totally lost control of everything. They no longer have meaningful personal relationships, because all the important people in their lives have likely left them. They may have lost their job and are probably experiencing severe financial problems. This is also the stage where excess drinking has caused enough health problems that the person's health has begun to seriously fail. At this point, if the person wants to quit drinking, they will definitely require professional assistance. If they do not drink, they will experience symptoms of withdrawal that might include sleep issues, irritability, nausea, profuse sweating, and tremors. The person may experience hallucinations or delusional thinking.

But where does alcoholism come from? The answers to that are extremely varied. While alcohol addiction begins with the act of drinking, many different factors will cause a person to tend towards becoming an alcoholic.

Sometimes drinking to excess is a family habit. There are those families that always have alcohol at every family function. Any excuse is a good excuse to have a drink. These families often have an addiction to other things too. They may overeat, overdo competition in sports, or constantly strive to be better than every other family on the block. People usually do not have just one addiction; people usually have addictive personalities and alcohol is the drug of choice.

Stress can cause people to drink excessively. Often people will take a drink in order to relieve the stresses of the day. In the early stages of alcohol addiction, people discover that a few social drinks will wash away the cares of the day. A little alcohol makes everything look and feel better. They remember this feeling and, when they have had a bad day, they take a drink or two just to 'take the edge off things.' Soon they are taking a few drinks whenever they have a bad day. Then a few drinks lead to a few more drinks.
Drinking to ease stress levels and drinking to self-medicate go hand in hand. Taking a few drinks to relieve the daily stress is one way to self-medicate. Sometimes people drink to hide the pain from a physical injury. More commonly people drink to hide the pain from an emotional hurt. People drink to dull the pain they feel when a loved one dies. People drink to erase the pain of a love that has gone wrong. People drink to hide feelings of inadequacy in social situation. Sometimes people drink to hide the pain from some sort of abuse or neglect.

And some people will drink to cover up the failures they feel in life. People who were turned down for a promotion, people who otherwise hate their professional life, those who cannot stand their family life—these are all people who drink to cover up the failures of life they have experienced. Their lives have not turned out as they hoped, so they drink to feel better about themselves.

Alcoholism begins quietly and attacks without warning. It can begin innocently, with one or two drinks, until the day it turns into an evil monster that takes over life.

Chapter 3: The Enabler

Most alcoholics would not remain alcoholics very long without the assistance of an enabler. The enabler helps the alcoholic hide their addiction from the world. The enabler is the person who faces all the bad things about alcoholism so the alcoholic can continue to pretend that there is nothing wrong with their drinking, that no real problem exists in their world.

The enabler is not willing to admit that there is a problem with the alcoholic. They will either overlook the existence of the problem or pretend that the problem does not exist, that it is all in someone else's mind.

To the enabler, the addict is never the person at fault. The problem lies with everyone else. Either the boss was too hard, the job was too demanding, the kids are too noisy, traffic was bad—the problem is never the fault of the addict and always the fault of anything or anyone else.

Fear is often a great motivator for the enabler. Often addicts act irrationally or angrily. They may blame all of life's problems on the enabler. Their behavior is often so frightening that the enabler will go to any length possible to avoid situations where the alcoholic will have reason to find fault with them.

The enabler will lie about anything and everything. The enabler will lie to the alcoholic's boss and claim they are sick yet again. The enabler will pretend extenuating circumstances are preventing them from coming to yet another family function or gathering of friends. They will always put the blame on themselves.

The addict will always come first in the eyes of the enabler. In the life of the enabler, the addict's needs will always be more important, even if it means neglecting their own needs. While wanting to help loved ones is normal, the enabler takes it much farther than that.

Enablers often experience great difficulty in showing emotions. They often have problems showing their innermost feelings, especially if they think the addict will subject them to negative thoughts, words, or actions for doing so.

The enabler takes care of many basic functions for the alcoholic, so they avoid much of the negative aspects of being an addict. The enabler will always make sure that there is enough of the right kind of alcohol in the house. The enabler will clean up any messes that the enabler makes, whether it is breaking a lamp in a drunken stagger through the house or even vomiting while intoxicated. The enabler will lie to others and make excuses for the alcoholic, even going so far as to take all the blame for the situation themselves. And the enabler will endure abject abuse from the alcoholic so that no one else will need to suffer their abuse. The enabler goes out of their way to make the situation seem better than it really is so that the alcoholic feels free to continue their downward spiral.

Chapter 4: Choosing to Quit Drinking and Its Benefits

Alcohol is everywhere. Just like food, it is an item often found at family gatherings, social events, and just about any kind of celebration imaginable. Many people use alcohol to cope with life's events. People drink to celebrate the arrival of new babies and the passing of loved ones. Alcohol is used to celebrate achievements and mourn over failures. And do not forget happy hour and the weekend.

Since alcohol and its use are so prevalent in today's society, making the decision to quit is not always easy. It can be a struggle for anyone, even the person with the greatest personal determination. When an alcoholic decides to quit drinking it is not a temporary decision, like a new diet or training for a marathon. When an alcoholic stops drinking it must be a lifelong decision. What makes a person an alcoholic is the inability to control their own drinking, to regulate the amount of alcohol consumed and how often it is consumed. For an alcoholic to be successful when quitting drinking they must never take another alcoholic drink ever again, not even one drop. This in itself can be a daunting task.

Changing any habit requires hard work, and drinking is a habit. Many people do not succeed the first time they decide to quit drinking, because drinking is not just a bad habit. Alcohol causes physical changes in the body that must also be addressed if quitting is to be successful. Failure is common, but it is not the end. Learn from failure and try again. Every try will be another step toward the goal. And if one method of quitting does not work, then try another method.

For someone to quit drinking alcohol requires a personal decision. No one can decide that another person should quit drinking. Even if the alcoholic is an underage person, they will not quit drinking just because they are told to. Love will not make someone else quit drinking. Neither will threats, tears, promises or even leaving them to their own devices. The alcoholic must make the decision because the path to sobriety is mainly a solo trip.

The alcoholic will not completely quit drinking until they are able to accept that they have a problem and want to change. The alcoholic does not care about lost jobs or lost family. They will simply drown their sorrows in another drink. They do not care if their friends abandon them because their one true friend, the bottle, is still there. The bottle never tells them they are a failure. The bottle never tells them the relationship is over or that they are no longer welcome here. The bottle loves them.

An alcoholic will not truly be ready to quit until they hit bottom, whatever their personal bottom is. The ultimate depth of failure is different for every person, and every person must hit that depth so they can go no lower. They must give up all their twisted notions of doing things their own way and be ready to accept outside help to curb this addiction. Because while the path to sobriety is a mostly personal path, it will require assistance from outside forces. And the alcoholic must be ready to accept this help in order to be successful. And they are the only ones who can make that decision.
If the decision to quit has been made that is the first step toward success. Tell everyone. Do not worry about what might happen if this goal is not successful. It might not be, but that is no reason not to try. Tell friends and family members that quitting drinking is the plan. Explain why the decision was made. People need to know and understand why personal habits have suddenly changed, why trips to the local bar or invitations out are suddenly being declined. Then people will be able to stop issuing those tempting invitations. And any little successes can be shared with everyone.

It will be best in the beginning to avoid all the places where drinking has historically occurred. This will also be a personal decision for the alcoholic to make. Favorite drinking spots are different for each person. It might be the local bar. It might be a favorite local restaurant. It will be necessary to avoid trivia night or the bowling league if those are occasions to drink. Any place that has ever been a place to go to consume alcohol must now be studiously avoided in order to remove possible temptation. In the beginning, the will power is too weak to simply think it is okay to go to familiar places and not drink.

Search past habits to see the particular times when drinking was more likely to be a focus. Is happy hour a problem? Is a liquid lunch a habit? Is it a regular practice to head to the bar on Friday or Saturday night after work? Write down all the times when having a drink would be a normal practice. This is especially important in order to be able to avoid these times. Drinking at a particular time is another habit that must be broken.

And definitely clear out all the little stashes of alcohol. Clean out the house. Search everywhere there might be some alcohol stashed. Ask others to help search if needed. It will be important to get all traces of alcohol out of the house before quitting.

Again, drinking is a habit that causes physical changes. Because of the physical changes, it causes it may be more difficult to stop drinking than to end other bad habits. Alcohol is a substance that causes addiction by activating the receptors in the brain that give pleasure. Every time these pathways are activated and give off pleasure signals, it gets harder and harder to get pleasure signals from these pathways. That is why alcohol is such a tough addiction to break because it has built to such a strong level over time.

So to quit drinking it will be necessary to not only make a mental decision but also to help the body support that decision physically. The body will need to be as strong as possible to fight this fight. After long term drinking, the body is probably malnourished and greatly in need of important nutrients. Start with frequent small meals of healthy nourishing foods. Proteins, fruits, and vegetables will become new best friends. Try to stay away from snack foods. These foods will not give the level of nutrition that the body needs right now, and the brain may associate them with drinking and start sending out cravings.

It might be helpful, before quitting, to make an effort to remove as much stress from everyday life as possible. Life itself is stressful and quitting drinking is even more stressful. If any of this stress can be removed, it will greatly increase chances of success. Set up direct deposit and automatic bill pay if possible. That will leave one less thing to worry about and will guarantee the bills get paid on time. Make weekly menus and prepare as much food as possible in advance. Clear space in the closet to line up a week's worth of clothing choices so it will only be necessary to grab that day's outfit and get dressed. Chose a gym buddy and set up a workout schedule. Any changes that can be made early will serve to remove much of the everyday decision making and allow focus to be spent on not drinking.

Be prepared to accept the physical symptoms that go along with quitting drinking. These are many and may include depression, excessive perspiration, sleep problems, shakiness, uneasiness, mood swings, and an increase in feelings of anxiety. These are what is known as withdrawal symptoms and can last anywhere from a few days to a few weeks. It just depends on how long the person has been drinking to excess.

And remember that this is a lifelong fight. This journey has no end. That is why people who quit drinking are called recovering alcoholic. Alcohol addiction is something that is always being recovered from. It will never be over. There is no cure.

But there are many benefits to quitting drinking. These include physical, mental, and emotional benefits as well a lifestyle and monetary changes.

Besides the obvious health changes—the clearer skin and eyes, stopping damage to the heart and liver—there are other health changes that are not often associated with drinking. Besides causing facial flushing excessive drinking can cause skin irritations like acne and eczema. The headaches that regularly follow a night of drinking will be a thing of the past. The dark circles under the eyes will gradually disappear. Sleep will come easier and will be deeper and more meaningful. Excessive consumption of alcohol causes malfunctions in a person's sex life, so quitting drinking will definitely lead to an improvement.

The excessive use of alcohol will cause an increase in anxiety and depression, even though people often turn to alcohol to deal with feelings of anxiety and depression. Once a person quits drinking these feelings will gradually return to a level where they can be more easily managed. Mood swings will gradually decrease. People who have quit drinking find they have better control over their everyday emotions. Granted they will need to learn other ways of coping with emotions besides drinking, but this will help lead to an overall better sense of self-worth.

People who quit drinking eventually find their mind is clearer and thoughts come easier. They forget things less than they did when they were drinking. They are better able to focus on the important things in life. Sober people are able to focus on the reason behind things and not look at everything emotionally.

Besides alcohol dependency, there are other major health effects to be concerned with. Even if excessive drinking does not currently affect health, it can lead to diseases that do not appear until years later. Some of the damage done to major organs may not be able to be healed or reversed. Structural changes in the brain may be improved. Quitting drinking can also assist with reversing the effects of alcohol on attention span, memory, and thinking ability, all of which alcohol affects negatively.

The decision to quit drinking must be a purely personal decision for purely personal reasons. No one became an alcoholic overnight, and no one can hope to be better overnight. It will take hard work and discipline. It will almost certainly be necessary to ask for outside help; in fact, sometimes the more help one has, the better their recovery will be. The road will not be easy, and failure will most certainly happen. But the rewards are too great to ignore.

Chapter 5: Best Method to Stop Drinking

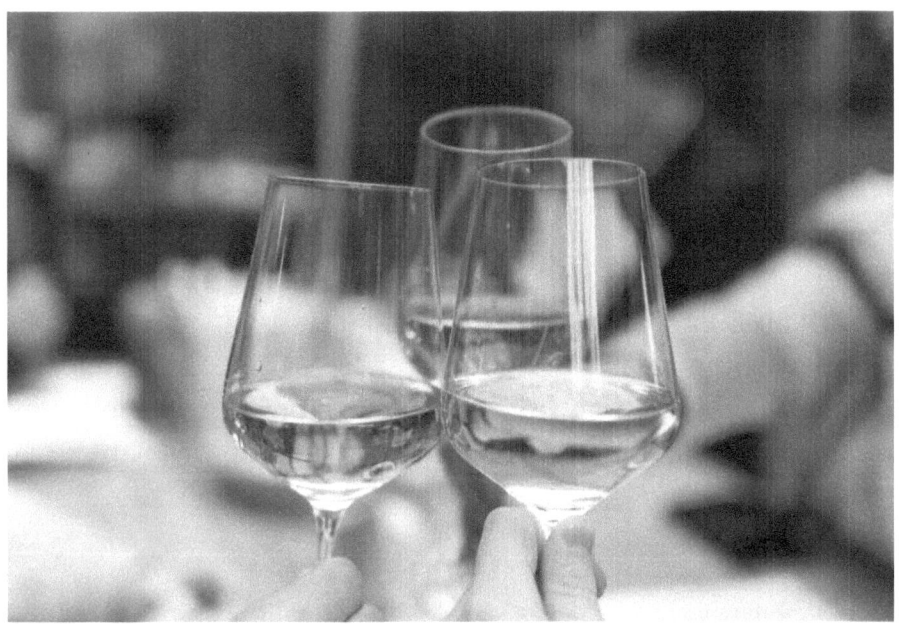

Anyone who seriously thinks they might have a serious drinking problem probably does. So instead of asking that question, ask if drinking is causing a problem with the enjoyment of everyday life. Ask exactly what effect alcohol is having on maintaining relationships. These questions will give insights to the problems currently being faced. No one should ever compare their own level and style of alcohol consumption to anyone else. Every addiction is personal just like every journey to sobriety will be personal.

Once the decision has been made to stop drinking it is important to list all the reasons that exist to stop drinking and accept them. No problem can be properly addressed unless it is accepted for what it is. Accept that an alcohol addiction exists and must be conquered in order to live a longer, more fulfilling life.

So how does one quit drinking? Well, the obvious answer is to stop buying alcoholic beverages and never drink another drop of anything alcoholic. That is basically what happens when someone quits drinking. But many different methods can be successfully used to help someone beat the pains of alcoholism.

One method that many people try, and many more think of trying, is a gradual decrease in the amount of alcohol that is consumed. Using this method will greatly decrease the possibility of suffering from alcohol-related withdrawal symptoms. Some of the symptoms that go along with suddenly quitting drinking are sleep disturbances, excessive sweating, tremors, headaches, anxiety, and depression. The idea behind gradually decreasing consumption is to hopefully lessen or eliminate these symptoms. These symptoms can possibly be quite severe, so attempting to quit drinking or at least to cut down on one's own without medical assistance would make tapering off a better option.

The easiest way to cut down on alcohol consumption is to reduce the actual number of alcoholic drinks consumed daily. This system is easy enough to follow. If the normal number of drinks taken daily is ten, then cut that down to eight for a while. How long it will take to feel more normal at the reduced level depends mostly on how many withdrawal symptoms are experienced and to what degree of severity. It may take several days for the withdrawal symptoms to cease. Then cut down the number of drinks again.

Other methods of tapering off include putting a greater amount of time in between individual drinks. If one drink each hour is normal, then drink one drink every two hours. Some people may stick to the one drink per hour schedule, but every other drink is water or a sports drink. Some people will alternate the every-other-hour drink with an alcoholic beverage they do not like the taste of, with the idea they will not drink a drink they do not like.

Tapering off is not a forever process. It needs to have an end date. So before beginning a system of cutting down on alcohol consumption, the most important part is to set an exact schedule the tapering off will follow along with a set date to stop drinking completely. And tapering off will not work for everyone with an alcohol addiction. Cutting down on the amount of alcohol consumed simply does not work for everyone, and it is nowhere near as effective a method for quitting alcohol as it is with other substances. Tapering off simply works better with nicotine or prescription drugs. Those who fail with this method are usually long term drinkers or those who can be considered heavy drinkers. It is also usually not successful for people who lack some sort of outside support system or are surrounded constantly by the triggers that led to alcohol addiction.

Doing a detox at home is not the best method for beating an addiction to alcohol. It may only be successful for those who have not been drinking long enough to form a strong addiction. It is a less expensive option and may work for those people who are not yet struggling with the negative effects of alcohol addiction.

Some medications are approved for treating alcohol addiction. One of these medicines is disulfiram, which is also known as Antabuse. It was the drug first approved by the FDA for use in individuals with alcohol addiction. Antabuse changes the chemistry inside the body to make people become violently ill if they drink an alcoholic beverage. It will work for people who are motivated to take it regularly. The problem is that people may have trouble taking a drug they know will cause the symptoms of a really awful hangover—sweating, vomiting, and headaches. But it does work when taken daily. It might also be appropriate for people who only feel the need to take a medication to counteract times they may be tempted to cheat.

Another medication that might be used for the treatment of alcohol addiction is the drug naltrexone. This drug works by suppressing the good feelings that come with drinking. So people can drink when they take naltrexone, and they will feel drunk, but they will not feel any of the good feelings generally associated with drinking. This medication can also help keep cravings at bay also. Usually when the alcoholic thinks about drinking the brain sends out feelings of pleasure. With naltrexone, these feelings are suppressed. This drug generally works best with someone who has already quit drinking.

Acamprosate, also known as Campral, is effective in relieving the symptoms of withdrawal that come with quitting drinking. Since withdrawal symptoms might last for many months after quitting drinking this drug can be an important part of recovery. The biggest drawback to Campral is the dosage amount. It usually requires taking two pills three or four times daily. This would not work for someone who is bad at remembering to take pills or does not like taking pills regularly.

Since alcohol has been around since the dawn of time, alcohol addiction has also been around that long. Before the last hundred years or so there was only one way known to man to quit drinking, and that was to go 'cold turkey,' to completely quit drinking any form of alcohol immediately, without the benefit of medication or tapering. Cold turkey is still in use today. But quitting drinking cold turkey should never be attempted without the supervision of a medical professional. Many alcoholics who stop drinking will suffer from severe symptoms of withdrawal including grand mal seizures from the convulsions and confusion of a severe level. These people may also suffer from cardiac arrhythmias and fevers that are dangerously high. People who have drunk excessive amounts over a long period are more likely to be affected by the most severe withdrawal symptoms. Also, consider that people who have been addicted to alcohol for a long time are most like undernourished and may not have the energy reserves to fight off the withdrawal symptoms effectively. And severe dehydration may affect people who are withdrawing from alcohol abuse. This can lead to a massive imbalance of electrolytes in the body that could lead to extreme confusion and a malfunction of the nerves and their responses.

Perhaps the most widely used method to quit drinking is the use of rehabilitation and detoxification. This is done during an in-patient setting at a medical facility. This method can be time-consuming and expensive, but it may be the only method that truly works for people with a deeply ingrained addiction. The level of care will depend greatly on the level of addiction.

Entering a treatment center for alcohol addiction is a totally voluntary decision. While entering treatment may be mandatory as part of a court sentence, it is still mainly a voluntary decision. The alcoholic must decide to go to treatment. Rehabilitation (rehab) centers are not like going to jail. There are no locks on the doors. The patient can leave at any time they chose to. There are house rules, and one of these rules is that continued alcohol and/or drug use will not be tolerated.

Some rehab facilities will offer detox services, and others will require that detoxing is done before entering the facility. Detox, or detoxification, refers to the process of cleansing the body of its immediate need for regular consumption of alcohol. Detoxing is the step number one in treating alcohol addiction. This is the time when alcohol is flushed completely out of the body. This is also when the symptoms of withdrawal will begin. As the body intakes less alcohol is will begin to suffer the ill effects of quitting. These symptoms generally stop within the first week or two but may end faster or last much longer depending on the level of addiction. These symptoms often make people fear to quit drinking because of the fear of these symptoms. That is why detox should be done under the care of a medical professional and possibly in a treatment center.

Once the worst symptoms of detox have passed, the alcoholic is ready to enter a treatment facility. These facilities are residential, meaning the person will live there for the duration of the initial treatment period. Treatment will fall into several phases but the first phase, the most intense, will be conducted on an in-patient basis. Rehab facilities vary in design from strict boot-camp style housing to something that more closely resembles a five-star hotel. The difference depends on the amount of money the patient can spend and what type of treatment they personally prefer. Keep in mind that the beauty or lack thereof in the facility has almost nothing to do with how successful they will be in making and keeping someone sober.

All rehab centers share one common trait: a severe lack of personal privacy. The patient will bring their own clothing and toiletries, but upon arrival, their bag will be checked for hidden sources of alcohol. Personal cell phones, laptops, and tablets usually are not allowed. There will be no contact with the outside world for at least two weeks. The idea is to make a complete break with the world the alcoholic could not function in and open up their minds to the possibility of a different way of life.

The basic component of all rehab centers is education. While the process will vary between facilities, it is all about getting people to take a more realistic and honest view of their personal addiction. They will also work to help the patient carefully examine the way they view alcohol use. During the early days of rehab, the vast majority of alcoholics will still hold on to some level of denial about how serious their problem really is. They may also be unsure of the fact that they really do have a problem. They may be denying that there is a problem, insisting they do not belong in rehab.

Classes in rehab will focus on alcoholism and its negative effects. One of the hardest things for alcoholics to accept is that they are suffering from a disease. It is difficult for people to believe that something that began as a socially accepted activity has turned into a disease. And a large part of the problem in treating alcohol addiction is that while individuals with alcohol addiction are held responsible for their actions they are usually not able to withstand the power of the alcohol that makes them act the way they do. So the patient will learn ways to counteract the mental effects of alcohol. They will also spend time learning what consequences they will face if they continue to use alcohol.

Rehabilitation makes use of group therapy and individual counseling. Group therapy will depend heavily on the individual's ability to talk about their problems in public. While the reason they are in rehab is probably similar to the reason everyone else is there, each patient will have a distinctly different back story. Everyone's path to alcohol addiction is different, just as everyone's path to sobriety will be quite different. The purpose of group therapy is twofold: point out dishonesty and assist with those who really want to succeed. Groups in group therapy are usually made up of patients in different levels of recovery and perhaps even some who have already graduated from inpatient therapy. They will be quick to point out when an addict is not completely honest about the nature of their addiction. People who cannot be honest about their addiction cannot possibly hope to recover. Group members are also quite willing to help those who really want help. And the patients learn to accept help from others who have gone before.

Individual counseling may also be part of the program. Some individuals will benefit greatly from the opportunity to have one-on-one counseling sessions with a personal counselor. The patient may feel some problems are too intense to share in group therapy, or they may have a series of deeply buried problems that need the guiding help a personal therapist can give. The individual counseling sessions may sometimes include family members. This is especially important since the patient will not have a meaningful recovery without the help and guidance of close family members and friends. And most rehab programs will require family members' attendance at counseling sessions apart from those with the patient.

An average day in a rehab facility begins with waking early for a hearty, healthy breakfast in the patient's dining room. Meals are not served in the room like in a hospital. Then there will be meditation groups, counseling groups, yoga, or some physical activity. After returning to the dining room for lunch, there will be more counseling with an emphasis on group sessions or family sessions. Late afternoon might see more physical activity, always some group activity like walking together on a trail or joining in a sport. Then, after a healthy dinner, it is time for shower and sleep. The entire schedule is designed to create a highly structured schedule for the patient, mainly so they can learn how to get structure back into their daily lives and so they can learn to take instructions from others. This will be especially important for the time following in-patient rehab.

The inpatient portion usually lasts four to eight weeks, depending on the facility and the level of treatment the patient requires, although some intensive programs can last up to one year. During the inpatient phase, the patient will learn many things about their addiction. They will also have learned how to take instructions from others regarding their addiction and will have learned how to depend on others for assistance in defeating their addiction. They will have learned to ask for help when they need it. This is especially important for the next phase of care where they will be back out in the world and will need to rely on outpatient plans.

After completing the in-patient part of the rehabilitation process, the patient is ready to leave the facility and begin outpatient therapy. This part of the program is especially critical, and it is where many fail, at least on the first try, because they are back in the real world without specialized guidance. No one is telling them when to eat breakfast or make their bed or go to group meeting. Now is when the alcoholic truly begins to understand living life without the alcohol crutch. Hopefully family and friends are there to lend support, but most of the burden falls on the alcoholic. And this is precisely why rehab is focused so heavily on the patient joining activities and speaking in group whether they wanted to or not. In the outside world, the patient needs to be able to ask for help when they need it.

No matter what method of quitting drinking is used, some form of counseling will be part of the process. This might mean that the patient continues to see a counselor for individual and/or group session. There will be separate family counseling for the family of the alcoholic, and there will be group counseling with the alcoholic and the family involved.

The counselor who assists alcohol addicted persons will know that everyone's recovery process is different. Each patient is a unique individual who will need a treatment plan geared specifically toward that individual. In the first few months following treatment at the rehab center the meeting with the counselor will be frequent, as many as four or five a week if needed. These meetings are important to help the recovering alcoholic stay on the right path. And the counselor, or a trusted colleague, will always be available by phone if a strong urge comes up during an off-meeting time.

The alcohol counselor will take an in-depth history of the patient's personal struggles with alcohol, and it is important the patient leaves nothing out. The more information the counselor has, the better the treatment plan will be. The counselor will set a plan for the patient's individual recovery, a sort of schedule of milestones the counselor hopes to achieve. They will discuss, in great detail, the things that led the patient to seek the comfort of alcohol in the first place. Because, after all, alcohol is a comfort, a coping mechanism, and ways to find the same comfort without drinking must be taught to the alcoholic. The counselor will also provide periodic assessments of progress and may reorganize the treatment plan if needed.

Recovery is not impossible, but it is a lifelong process that will require strict attention and much hard work. But, once abstinence becomes a way of life, the personal rewards are endless.

Chapter 6: Kill the Cravings

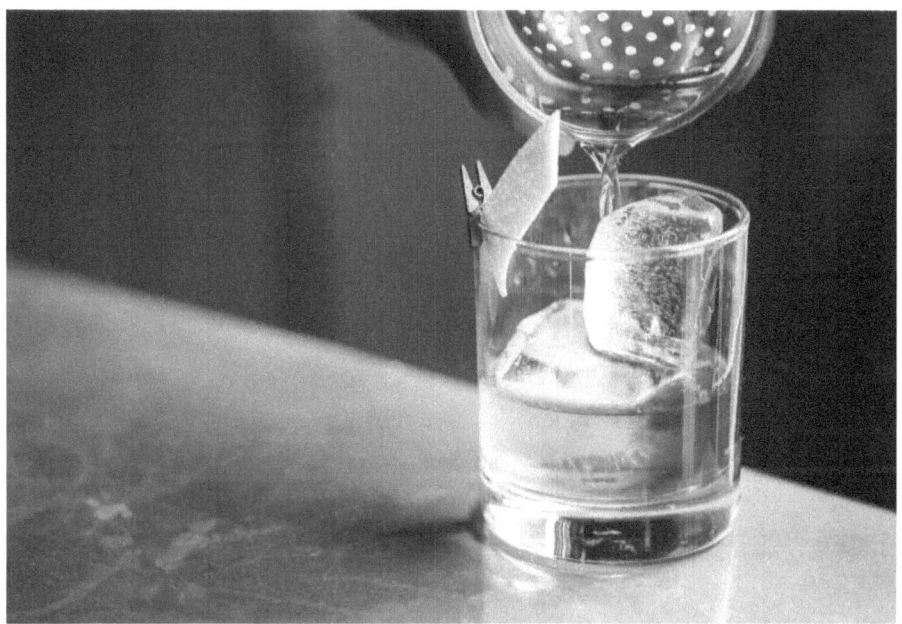

Once the alcoholic has embarked on a life of sobriety, there should be no more consumption of alcohol, ever. Remember an alcoholic is always in recovery, and even one drink can send a person back down the spiral into alcoholism. So it is important to abstain from drinking forever.

Unfortunately, the cravings still exist. A craving is a strong mental or physical urge to eat or drink something. A craving pulls a person's thoughts in one direction only, and the focus is this thing that must be consumed. If the alcoholic gives in to these cravings for alcohol, they will be right back where they started.

These cravings, or urges, are usually controllable with a little planning and effort. After time urges will gradually lessen. This is because new pathways of information have been laid out in the brain. Where before the craving would send a message to tell the body to drink, now when the craving hits the body sends back the confusing message that it is going to do something other than drink alcohol. At first, the mind will be quite confused. But with time those old pathways will be shut down and replaced with new pathways and the urges to drink will begin to subside.

There are two types of events that can cause an urge to drink. These are called 'triggers.' The triggers that are external come from everyday life and the things, places, people, and events that make up the external world. The other type of trigger is internal and may be more confusing, and therefore harder to control, to the recovering alcoholic.

Triggers caused by external events can sometimes be relatively easy to control. If the daily happy hour was formerly a time to drink, then happy hour will not be a future destination. If the weekend barbeques overflowed with beer, then the beer needs to be left in the store. The trick is to either reprogram the mind to enjoy certain events alcohol-free or to avoid those events altogether. Sometimes people cause a trigger. The boss is being unreasonable, so a quick nip is in order. This may be the time to decide if the boss is being unreasonable or if the problem is really internal. If friends want to go on a pub crawl, the answer is certainly 'no.' This will likely mean changing old habits and losing old friends, but it is vital to the recovery process.

Triggers that come from within can be harder to figure out because there is no obvious event to place the blame on. The urge to have a drink just seems to appear out of nowhere. These urges will need to be examined in great detail by the recovering alcoholic, perhaps with the help of his counselor, to determine exactly what set off the urge to drink. For example, if before the alcoholic drank to ease the pain of a headache, then a headache caused by too much time in the sun might cause an urge to drink. This is the time for the alcoholic to be completely honest with themselves and overlook nothing, no matter how trivial it might seem.

The counselor will be available for those times when a craving cannot be ignored. And there will be other groups that will assist the alcoholic on the path to recovery.

It might also help to engage in something the person used to love doing or to learn something new. This might be a good time to reconnect with a love of art or keeping a journal. A journal is an especially good idea because the patient can write down anything they think or feel and it is completely private until they chose to share it. Maybe the person used to play volleyball or weekend pickup games of basketball at the neighborhood park. Get back to doing the activities that once brought happiness to life. It might be time to try something new. Recovery is all about breaking out of old habits and forming new ones. Maybe it's time to try ballroom dancing or poetry reading. A new high-risk skill might be in order too. Since alcoholics crave the rush that alcohol brings, maybe that rush could be found elsewhere, perhaps with skiing or boxing.

The possibilities are endless. The important thing is to realize that this is the path to a new more meaningful life and the script has not been written. This phase of life can be anything the recovering alcoholic wants it to be and now is the time to take advantage of that opportunity.

Chapter 7: Change Thoughts and Mindset

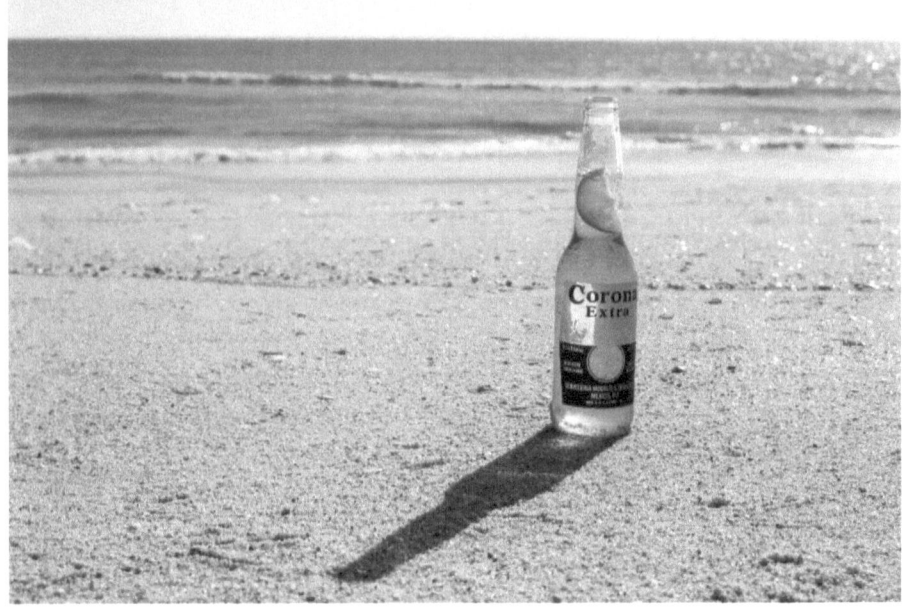

Now is the time for a whole new mindset. Remember, this is all about starting life over. The past is gone because it cannot be changed anyway. It is now time to look forward, believing that every day is a new day and recovery is possible.

Beginning this new phase of life requires resetting processes in the mind. Remember, habits are formed when the mind lays down a nerve pathway to a particular spot in response to a constant stimulus. One simple example is learning to flip a pancake in the pan. By putting the flipper under the pancake and turning the wrist, the pancake should flip over to the other side for cooking. But this might not happen in the beginning. The nerve path has not been laid. During practice, the nerve pathway becomes stronger until it is finally set. So when the flipper is slid under the pancake, this is the stimulus that travels to a point in the brain that sends a message telling the wrist to turn is a specific way in order to turn the pancake over in the pan. It sounds complicated, but this is what the mind does daily, and the mind is very good at it.

The activities and behaviors that the patient engages in after rehab are much like this. When a routine is practiced often, the mind develops very deep pathways with a thin layer of insulation surrounding them. This is to allow the signal to travel faster and easier. And just like current habits are easy to perform, new activities and behaviors will eventually become habits.

The mind is a powerful tool on the path to sobriety. The first step to creating new mind paths is to acknowledge the existence of the old ones. Pay particular attention to negative thoughts that will put mental blocks in the path to recovery. Change negative thoughts into positive ones. You do deserve this new life. You are strong enough to achieve this goal. You will remain sober. In the beginning, the mind may try to negate these thoughts. It's sort of like the good angel and the bad angel sitting on one's shoulder. Do not let the bad angel win.

The recovering alcoholic may be forced to find new places to go where alcohol will not be a temptation. Obviously, the bar is now off limits because the temptation will be too great. Even walking in the door and smelling the alcohol in the floating haze will be enough of a trigger to bring back the drinking. But what about other places where alcohol might be served? If the function is at home, then make it alcohol-free. You can do what you want in your own house. Do not serve alcohol, and make it very clear during the invitation process that no alcohol will be allowed on the premises. The home is a personal safe space and should be kept safe. But think about events like concerts and sporting events, where alcohol is served. If the path to the seat can be routed somewhere other than right past the alcohol vendors, that would be a good thing. Maybe the plan is to go to the seat first and let someone else go for refreshments. If there is no viable option, then it may be necessary to avoid these events, at least in the beginning when resistance might still be weak.

Unfortunately the recovering alcoholic will likely be forced to find a new set of friends. The old friends who still go on pub crawls and weekend binges will not understand this new sober lifestyle. Hanging out with them just increases the urges to drink and the possibility that a relapse can occur. So as much as it might hurt in the beginning, it might be better to leave them behind. But turn this into a positive by thinking of the rewards offered by this new lifestyle. Not only is alcohol a thing of the past, opening up a whole new future, but there are so many new people to be discovered. Whether these new friends come from the rehab center, group therapy, church, scheduled meetings, or new hobbies discovered, the possibilities are endless. The chance to make so many new friends will make life feel exciting and new.

Chapter 8: Recovery Plan

One of the most important parts of alcohol recovery is to have a plan in place to facilitate that recovery. No goal is ever reached without a plan. The key is knowing what to do next, so there is little to no room for error when the alcoholic reenters the real world outside of rehab. This plan will contain goals and activities that will give the recovering alcoholic guidance for coping with the outside world.

The recovery plan needs to be set up by the recovering alcoholic because it is their plan. It is personal to them. It will list everything they need to know and to do to get started on the path to recovery and stay on track.

One important part of the plan will include those things that make the alcoholic feel better, those things that lead to a feeling of wellness. These are simple things, events no more complicated than quiet time at home, exercising, family time, walks in the park, reading, or soaking in the bathtub. The list will consist of simple, no-cost activities that can be done without much travel or complexity. These are the things that make the person feel good inside, and these activities will be used to replace the old activities that led to drinking. Review these items at least daily, more often if it helps make the path to sobriety easier to walk. These activities will bring about positive thoughts that will help erase the negative thoughts that led to excessive drinking.

Make a list of known triggers. Make this list as comprehensive as possible. Most alcoholics know those events that will set off the cravings for alcohol. Be brutally honest. If the kids' screaming happily while playing is a trigger, then write that down, it can be addressed and acted upon as needed. The key is to list everything. This is where the alcoholic will discover those things that cause cravings so that a plan can be put into place to either avoid these events or to fix them if they cannot be avoided completely. Going to the local bar can be avoided. Stress at work cannot be avoided.

The alcoholic must know and list their own personal warning signs that the cravings are about to take over the common sense. Only be recognizing these triggers can a person hope to defend against them. Again, write them down and be brutally honest. They cannot be fixed if they are not known. If being isolated from other people causes feeling of cravings then perhaps regular trips to the park, a cultural event, or even church will make the person feel less isolated and more a part of society. If being irritable or angry triggers desires to drink then a new coping mechanism must be determined as it is nearly impossible to go through life and never be angry or irritated. Perhaps the strategy here would include a few minutes of quiet meditation or a brisk walk around the block. Whatever the coping strategies are they must be personal and actionable. And if a particular strategy does not work, then change it.

And since major crises will happen in everyone's life, a plan must be in place to help the recovering alcoholic cope with crises. These fall into two categories: the ones that the individual can handle with someone else's assistance and the ones where the individual has totally lost control.

If the problem is one that the alcoholic can handle with assistance, then there are numerous resources at their disposal. It then is simply a matter of reaching out for help. Certainly, the alcoholic should be able to turn to family members to help them get through an intense craving or major life event. Sometimes greater help is needed. This would be the time when a person would turn to their personal counselor to talk to while trying to cope. They may have kept in touch with other patients from the rehab center. If so then now is the time to call them. They understand better than anyone the struggle the alcoholic is facing and would be well equipped to helping them cope. A buddy from a support group is another option. They are tasked with helping their partner on their travels toward sobriety, just as someone gives them the same type of assistance.

There may be times when the recovering alcoholic is beyond private help and must be referred to a professional. A relapse into drinking is one of these times, certainly, but there are others not related to actual drinking. The person may have become extremely agitated or violent over some happening and may need a visit to the doctor or a medical facility. The important thing is to recognize the possibility of these behaviors before they happen and to decide at what point outside intervention is needed.

Once this plan is set, take a few minutes each day to revisit the plan and to reflect on any successes for the day. Acknowledge any small failures but do not dwell on them. One of the goals is to replace negative thoughts with positive thoughts, so try to keep this activity as positive as possible.

Decide whether addiction is the biggest problem or if other problems in life are bigger. It may be that drinking is the one big problem in life. Some people drink to excess simply to drink to excess. They are not trying to cover up underlying problems or cope with life; they just drink too much because it is there to drink. These people will need to focus mainly on avoiding taking that next drink. But most people drink because they need to cope with life. These people will need to focus on ways to deal with the events and problems that crop up in everyday life that might cause the person to want to drink to excess again.

Remember that cravings can be controlled. Cravings are nothing more than a message the brain sends in response to a particular stimulus. Cravings do not last forever. Cravings will not kill a person, although it may feel like it at the time. And cravings cannot make anyone do anything they do not want to do. The choice is up to the individual.

Be ready to engage in a lifelong marathon. This is not a quick race. This will take forever, at least however long a person's forever is. An alcoholic who no longer drinks is recovering, always recovering. There is no cure to alcoholism.

There are outside forces that can help the recovering alcoholic on their way to recovery. Anyone who has ever had an addiction to alcohol and been successful in overcoming it will recommend taking advantage of one or more of these options to ensure the goal of sobriety is reached.

Of course, total abstinence must be observed. The recovering alcoholic must never drink again if they want to continue recovering. Even a drop of alcohol would be enough to trigger a relapse into mindless drinking. They must not have alcohol in the house or go to places alcohol will be served. This is especially important in the early days when will power is weak.

After leaving the rehabilitation center, there is always the possibility of returning. Especially in the beginning, some people feel the need for a refresher course, or they may feel as though they left the rehab facility before they were really ready. There is nothing wrong with this decision. The important thing is to do whatever needs to be done to help the addict recover.

Ongoing counseling is very important. The breakthroughs that happened while in rehab need to continue. More work needs to be done on triggers and cravings, and goals and achievements. There is no end to this journey; it is for life.

Never overlook the power of the buddy system. Having a buddy is crucial to recovery for the alcoholic. The buddy is the one person the addict can call who will always answer the phone, day or night. Living life as a sober person is difficult. A buddy is someone set up by the support group to be personally responsible for the sobriety of another person. This buddy must have shown that they have been sober for quite a while and are comfortable helping someone else to reach sobriety. This sponsor is responsible for doing everything they can to help another person not drink alcohol. They must always lead by example and encourage their buddy to attend as many meanings as possible. They guide their sponsee through the requirements of the group and what to do to be successful in sobriety. And, perhaps most importantly, they will answer the phone whenever their sponsee calls needing help in getting past that potentially fatal craving.

No discussion of alcohol addiction recovery would be complete without mentioning Alcoholics Anonymous (AA). AA was founded many years ago by two men who wanted a structured method to use to quit drinking. The program was based on using spiritual growth to achieve character development. One way to develop a good character was to refrain from drinking. They also developed the program of twelve steps that lead the practitioner to the ultimate goal of sobriety.

The policy of following the prescribed steps is crucial to success in AA. These steps are needed to ensure potential success. The addict must be able to accept that they have no power over alcohol but that it has much power over them. They need to believe in some sort of higher power of their choosing and to give their lives to the control of that higher power. They must be able to admit they have made mistakes and to own their mistakes. They must be willing to confront those people who have contributed to their addiction and to apologize to those they have hurt with their actions. And they must continually work through the process as the path to the goal changes because life changes.

The only definite requirement for joining an AA meeting is a fervent wish to live a sober life. AA accepts everyone whether rich or poor, regardless of race, creed, religion, origin, or anything else that might exclude someone from a group. In group meetings, only first names are used. This helps people feel that they can be totally open and honest about their past histories without giving up too much identifying information. And there is no age restriction for group meetings since alcoholism can strike at any age. One meeting a week is a bare minimum; people are encouraged to attend several meetings each week whenever possible. And everyone is encouraged to have a home meeting group where they go regularly, but it is an easy matter to find a group to join almost anywhere that the addict might be traveling for business or pleasure. The idea here is that there is always a group available for help. And it is during an AA meeting that one would be assigned a sponsor, that buddy who will answer the phone whenever they call.

Along with AA, there are the groups Al-anon and Alateen. Al-anon is a group for the friends and families of recovering alcoholics. Alcoholism is never a private disease. It affects everyone the alcoholic comes into contact with. Al-anon is a place these people can go to learn ways to cope, ways to help, and ways to forgive. Alateen does much the same thing, but it is specifically for young children and teens whose lives have been affected by someone who drinks, whether that person is currently in their lives or not. The alcoholic parent might still be present in the home. The alcoholic might be an absentee parent because of the alcoholism. Either way, the group will provide support when needed. Both groups offer the same type of sponsorship found in AA.

Setting oneself up for a good recovery is an important step on the road to recovery. The person who can leave alcohol addiction behind on their own is the rare person. Most people will need many levels of help before they can even begin to consider that sobriety might be a viable way of life. There is nothing wrong and everything right with being able to ask for help when it is needed. Remember this is a journey, and everyone needs help somewhere along the way. Just reach out and ask for it.

Chapter 9: The Role of Others in The Life of the Recovering Alcoholic

Addiction to any substance will affect everyone around the addict. People find it difficult to believe that anyone would prefer a drunken stupor to a life of sobriety. Keep in mind that alcoholism is a disease and must be treated as such. Someone who has a heart attack or a stroke will potentially have a long recovery period and will need support. The same is true of the alcoholic.

Every family group has a balance point. That is the point at which the family functions the best. This may not necessarily be a good function, but this is the way the family functions in this house. Every family is different, and the alcoholic's family is no exception to this rule.

The first problem the family might face after the alcoholic quits drinking is a shift in balance. The family life was settled around the care of the addict, and now that consideration has been removed. It can completely disrupt life as the family knows it and require a major rebalancing act to get back to normal. Keep in mind this is not the dictionary definition of normal but what is normal for the family.

Pretend the father is a raging alcoholic. The family has learned to walk on tiptoe when dad is home. No unnecessary noise is made in the house. Children tend to disappear, either to their rooms or somewhere outside, in order to avoid the wrath of dad. Mom might lie about problems the children might be having so that she will not incur dad's anger and the children will not suffer. When dad suddenly becomes sober and is no longer a raving lunatic the balance of the family has tilted. Dad might now want to have a relationship with the very children he has frightened so many times. Mom might not know how or when to share the children's activities with dad in the fear that he may go off the deep end again. The family will need to rebalance.

Suppose mom is the alcoholic. Mom is unable to do any of the things mommy usually does because she is always drinking or drunk. Dad and possible older children pick up the slack and do all the cooking, cleaning, and nurturing. Now suppose mom gets clean and comes home to resume her mommy life. She may be unable to because, for so long, she did none of these things. The children now turn to dad or older siblings for everything they need because mommy cannot be trusted to help them. The family will need to rebalance.

Whatever roles people play in the family, they need to expect that this new sobriety will cause changes in the family dynamic. In time these changes will be good ones that will serve to strengthen the family unit. Some adjustment will be needed to reach that point, but it is not impossible.

Chapter 10: The Dangers of Relapse

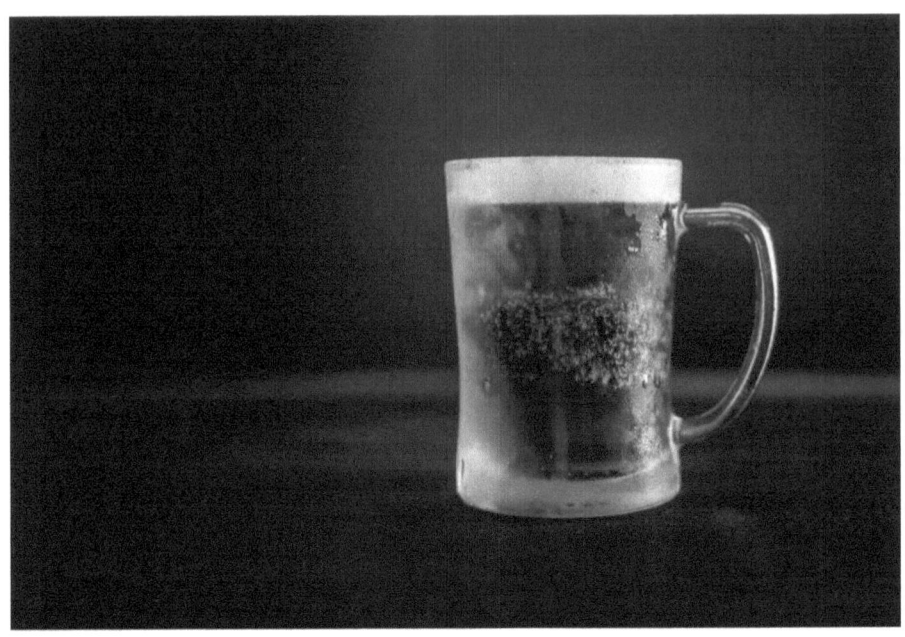

Long term sobriety is an achievable goal, with the right kind of work. Unfortunately, the level of support that is available in the early days is not the same level of support that will be available for the remainder of the addict's life. Eventually, it is understood that the person who is recovering has achieved a certain sense of self-worth and self-confidence and will be able to guide themselves, with minimal assistance, on their journey. This may not be the case for everyone. Some people enjoy a textbook recovery and rarely experience problems, but these people are very few and far between. Most people are quite human and become accustomed to a certain level of attention while they are recovering. When this attention is taken away, they may begin to falter.

Some specific signs signal that a relapse might be imminent. Cravings may begin to increase again. There may be thoughts of taking 'just one drink' just to get past a rough patch. The recovering alcoholic might feel abandoned or stuck in one place in their recovery. Feelings of depression and anxiety may return, worse than ever before. The addict may begin to deny his real feelings in favor of keeping the peace. They may begin to have an abnormal interest in other potentially harmful behaviors like gambling, overworking, overeating, or sexual experiencing. These new interests may become an addiction in themselves. These are mental reactions to a possible relapse that happen before the relapse occurs.

Next would be the physical reactions that will make the relapse more likely to happen. The physical part is more dangerous because it may involve an actual exposure to the very substance that caused a problem in the first place. This can include boredom with the current situation or fear that support may not be available when needed. Spending an inordinate amount of time talking about drinking is also a bad sign. There might be an actual feeling of physical pain that makes the addict think about drinking. There might be an increase in negative emotions like anxiety, sadness, and loneliness. Being around alcohol at this time would be particularly dangerous.

Again, the addict should never be afraid to ask for help. Just because the resources are no longer hovering does not mean that they are no longer available. The sponsor is still available anytime of the day or night. The members of the group are still there and ready to help. The counselor still has an office and is still ready to listen. When the addict regains some of their strength, this might be a good time to consider becoming a sponsor. Helping someone else along the path to sobriety is a wonderful way to renew one's own convictions in one's abilities.

Chapter 11: Pleasure Without Hangover

So the decision has been made, and the alcohol has been left behind. The addict has been through rehabilitation. The many counseling sessions have become the occasional visit. New friends have been made. Unfortunately, some old friends were lost along the way, but in the process of alcohol recovery that happens sometimes. The old hangouts are now off limits. The family is back together, and everyone seems to be enjoying the new dynamic. Work has never been better. What now?

Now is the time to learn to enjoy life without the bottle hanging around the neck like a big glass noose. Everything has now changed, most of it for the better, and it will continue to change for the positive as long as hard work and dedication are applied. Much of the early intense focus on remaining alcohol-free has relaxed and now it is time to get on with the business of enjoying life. But how?

There are a few truths about alcohol that no alcoholic will ever admit until after they quit drinking. Alcohol sneaks into a person's life under the guise of a friend, a helper. Alcohol will make everything better. Alcohol will make all the pain go away. Alcohol will make everything clear and sunny again. And in the beginning, it does just that. Drinking alcohol makes everything bigger and funnier. Life is so much better with alcohol.

Then alcohol begins to show its true colors, but the alcoholic cannot see these until they quit drinking. It is only then that they learn the dirty truth about alcohol.

Alcohol ends more fun than it starts. Constantly needing to find ways to work alcohol into the situation means missing out on a lot of fun. Think of all the parties never attended because alcohol was not offered. Think of all the children's plays and recitals missed or even gotten too late because of one more drink. The truth is that parties without alcohol are not dull; the dullness comes from the attendees who need alcohol to liven up and cannot function if it is not present.

Alcohol will steal from anyone it finds to steal from. Alcohol does not care. Alcohol will ruin a person's health. The longer someone drinks the more health problems they will experience. And some of these problems have no cure when they get to their worst stage: think heart attack, stroke, and a dead liver. Alcohol steals relationships and makes the alcoholic a lonely person. Alcohol steal time that could better be spent on anything else but is now lost forever. And alcohol steals money because alcohol in excess is very expensive.

If possible, the recovering alcoholic should watch other sober people in the process of getting drunk. They will be able to see their friends turn into bleary-eyed uncoordinated strangers. They will laugh at things that are not really funny. They will insist they are having a wonderful time when the smile on their faces does not reach their eyes. And tomorrow morning they will wake up with dry mouth and a hangover while trying to recall what really happened last night.

The real truth is that embracing sobriety is not so much about the end of a life and more about the beginning. Certainly, the party life must be left behind. But so much more of life is now open for the taking that it can sometimes feel unbelievable.

People who have started on a life of sobriety now have time to learn who they are and what they want out of life. There is no longer the consideration of needing a drink, or several, to be able to function. Now they can decide what they want out of all areas of life. Is the addict holding onto a particular job they do not like simply because the employer put up with him when he was drinking? If so it might be time for a career change. While it is nice if an employer stuck behind a person, that bond will not hold two people together forever. Decide what type of career is best and make a change if the time feels right.

Now is the time to enjoy family outings. Think of all the school plays, recitals, family picnics, holiday dinners, birthdays, that were missed because either alcohol was not being served or the addict was already too drunk to participate. There is no alcohol standing in the way anymore. Enjoy the family and spend some time mending fences. It will be well worth the work.

Did any hobbies get left behind in the search for the next drink? Or were some never attempted because they might interfere with drinking? Now is the time to pick up the brush and easel that has been collecting dust in the attic. That project car in the garage, the one that has been waiting under a tarp for years, could be the perfect vessel for reconnecting with the kids. Maybe the community center has been offering a pottery class for years that directly interfered with happy hour. Well, alcohol is now out of the picture, and now it is time to find a hobby or two to enrich life.

If the most horrible thing happened and late night drinking and driving resulted in the loss of a license and driving privileges, now is the time to work on getting them back. An approved alcohol awareness program is usually a requirement to regain a lost license. Someone already on the road to sobriety has already taken the necessary steps to becoming a sober driver and the courts like that. Get the license back and get out in the world again.

Sobriety will not always be easy. Never drinking again will sometimes be the hardest decision ever made. Twenty years in the clear might pass, and one horrible event might prompt a craving for a drink. This is a life-long journey that is worth so much to every area of life that it makes no sense not to start on the path. With hard work and dedication, the goal of sobriety can be reached.

Conclusion

Thank you for making it through to the end of *Alcohol Addiction: How to Stop Drinking and Recover from Alcohol Addiction*. Let's hope it was informative and able to provide you with all of the tools you need to achieve your goals whatever they may be.

The next step is to make the personal decision to stop drinking and just do it. This decision is difficult, this decision is scary, but it is probably the best decision you will ever make in your life. Because the decision to quit drinking will positively affect not only your life but the lives of friends and loved ones forever. Quitting drinking is a lifelong journey and the best time to start is now.

BONUS:

As a way of saying thank you for purchasing my book, please use your link below to claim your free ebook

I have laid down Top 10 Tips Guide for you to Overcoming Obsessions and Compulsions Using Mindfulness

https://bit.ly/2TDMNkn

You can also share your link with your friends and families whom you think that can benefit from the guide or you can forward them the link as a gift!

www.ingramcontent.com/pod-product-compliance
Lightning Source LLC
Chambersburg PA
CBHW030732180526
45157CB00008BA/3141